MURMURATION

MURMURATION

A.J. LEES

MIRABEAU PRESS

Published by Mirabeau Press

PO Box 4281

West Palm Beach, FL 33401

ISBN: 979-8-9939674-1-7

First Edition

MIRABEAU

CONTENTS

FOREWORD

Anyone who has been a patient of late — and, above a certain age, that is likely to include most people — will have noticed that medical practice has changed. A patient is more likely to be treated as a question asked of ChatGPT than he is as a living, thinking, feeling being.

I can attest to this myself. Usually of good health, I recently experienced a sudden brief episode of illness. It took me four algorithms — always the same one, but each time with a different conclusion, I suppose because each was designed to answer a different question and for a different end — to reach hospital. Finally, I was rushed there, siren blaring and light flashing, to wait nearly four hours outside in a traffic jam of ambulances. No history was taken, no physical examination performed. I had a blood test and a CT scan and waited an hour for a doctor to inform me that I was perfectly all right, apart from my blood pressure. After the four algorithms by telephone, no one, apart from the ambulance crew, had asked me anything or laid a finger on me. The doctor was with me for about three minutes at most.

It is against this kind of medicine that Andrew Lees, a

distinguished professor of neurology, eloquently protests in this book of aphorisms, the fruit of decades of experience and reflection. It is generally believed that knowledge and skill only accumulate and cannot be lost, but this is not the case. A generation of doctors who do not know how to take a history from patients or examine them, and do not even think it necessary to be able to do so, will not only be unable to pass the skills on to their own students when the time comes, but will have become at best auxiliaries to their machines, without the ability to think for themselves.

Professor Lees is not a detractor of modern technology: how could any man be who has made neurological research a large part of his life? But developments in medical practice seem not only to throw the baby out with the bathwater, but the bath as well. No doubt some of his observations in this book will seem recondite to non-neurologists, but the gist of this *cri de coeur* will be clear to everyone: if we dehumanise medicine, we dehumanise ourselves. Professor Lees' book is a contribution to halting that baleful process.

Theodore Dalrymple

INTRODUCTION

Murmuration does not refer to a swarm of starlings in a back end sky but to the way human beings can sometimes interconnect and produce spontaneous, imaginative social outcomes. I hang on to the illusory hope that this might one day return to Twitter. Since the publication of *Neurological Birdsong*, Elon Musk, the ultrarich entrepreneur, has bought the social media platform for 44 billion US dollars. In spite of his outlandish claim that his new algorithms are helping to defend democracy, many of the interesting strangers with whom I had once exchanged sparky ideas have bolted. Academics, too, left in their droves for more decentralised social networking sites like Mastodon and Bluesky. A close friend told me that staying on Twitter (rebranded now as 'X') was similar to buying and driving a Tesla car. After switching, I immediately missed the Twitter interchanges with mavericks and contrarians, investigative journalists, people with neurological disorders, and Northern soul survivors. Posting on Bluesky felt like blowing a euphonium alone in my front room.

As my winters get progressively longer and my springs less

vivid, the temptation to cause mischief intensifies. I enjoy giving anti-educational universities, the greedy 'private for-profit' medical industrial complex and uncritical colleagues some well-intentioned pokes in the eye. With advancing age, opportunities to get out more become fewer, and in any case, it is fun being a bloody nuisance. I am treated like an aging rock star whose voice has gone or a borderline national treasure when I attend the Gowers Grand Round at the National Hospital, Queen Square. On the rare occasions my opinion is asked, I am often relieved to find that basic clinical observations that were once familiar to all doctors are now sometimes greeted as awesome revelations.

I have drifted back to Twitter as a way of hanging on. In my head, I am a free-thinking rebel, defending the craft of neurology against the dark knights who stalk the medical industrial complex. I block evil trolls or bots and censor any hate material that appears unannounced on my screen. I refuse to subscribe to Premium X and have no desire to become the holder of a blue checkmark or write a 25000-word tweet. As with my first collection, my colleague Ibrahim Imam has helped to select and then collate the content. I am indebted to him and also to Mirabeau Press for publishing the book.

In the last two years, I have acquired even more bees in my bonnet, and as a consequence *Murmuration* may come over as a little more strident than *Neurological Birdsong*. Academic medicine particularly is in trouble, bedevilled by fraud, bias, red tape, stuck in set thinking and an unhealthy adoration and unshakeable belief in 'sexy' science. It is also suffering from a disease named jargon which interestingly, in relation to the titles of my books of tweets, is an Old French word translated as the chattering of birds.

This year, two separate publications in *Lancet Neurology* have proposed a biological definition of Parkinson's disease, based on the premise that accumulation of abnormally aggregated alpha synuclein in nerve cells is important in the causation of Parkinson's disease and the development of a new amplification seed assay, which measures the abnormal protein in human tissue. The companies responsible for marketing the test envisage it as an acid test tantamount to finding malignant cells in cancer, which will diagnose Parkinson's disease without the need to take a medical history or carry out a neurological examination. These inflated claims have led to controversy. My view is that all the authors of these papers have achieved so far is to recast healthy people as being sick and opened the door for the pharmaceutical industry to administer experimental treatments to people who may never develop Parkinson's disease.

I have also been critical of the over-egged claims for new immunological therapies for Alzheimer's disease that remove amyloid plaques from the brain. The improvements in cognition demonstrated in the trials with lecanemab and donanemab are slight and lead to a degree of improvement on rating scales that has previously been reported with brain training alone, such as doing a crossword puzzle every day. These new amyloid busting drugs are also very expensive (30,000 US dollars a year per patient) and carry a considerable risk of brain haemorrhage.

The study of nervous disorders requires a long apprenticeship, a respect for tradition and rituals, pride in one's work, and a lifelong commitment to and immersion in 'the thing itself'. Neurology is a practical art, not an applied science. I never stop being amazed at the progress that has occurred in my chosen craft. CT and MR head scanners have made neurological investigation quicker, safer and cheaper, and have improved the accuracy of diagnosis. Thrombolysis (clot busting) and endovascular recanalization can now sometimes avoid irreversible neurological impairment after a stroke. L-DOPA has improved the quality of life in Parkinson's disease, and immunological modulation has reduced the number of relapses in multiple sclerosis. There have also been advances in epilepsy surgery and the treatment of headache, while gene therapies for hereditary neurological disorders are starting to reach the bedside. Nevertheless, there is no room for complacency, especially in relation to the diagnosis and management of neurodegenerative disorders like Alzheimer's disease, motor neurone disease and the treatment of malignant brain tumours. In an article written in the Lancet in 1949, Dr Richard Asher listed the seven medical sins as: obscurity (relating to oral communication and writing), cruelty, bad manners, overspecialisation, love of the rare and exotic (Spanophilia), common stupidity and laziness. Only cruelty has clearly diminished since Asher's day. My own bugbears include technophilia (often associated with lack of basic clinical skills), cowardice, boosterism, a view that new is always better than old ('early advocates' of new treatments and tests), venality, disease-mongering and omniscience.

Soulful neurologists are curious about the lives of their patients as well as their diseases. They require a worldly wisdom, tacit knowledge, and sound judgement to practice their craft. Rather than jumping to conclusions or ordering tests without reflection, they listen, think, watch, and wait. They believe in 'the positive art of doing nothing' as a way of avoiding harm. In comparison to other branches of medicine, neurology has more known unknowns. It is important therefore that, as a speciality, we acknowledge our ignorance and try to find answers to the questions our patients ask and for which we have no answer. A few of the tweets express my faith in serendipity as an important route to medical discovery.

Many of the aphorisms in this book have their roots in the clinic, but I hope that my grumbling will resonate far beyond the confines of medicine. Health and medicine seem to be of endless fascination for the public, and after all even doctors and nurses are patients too.

A. J. Lees
The National Hospital, Queen Square, London

A. ACADEMIC MEDICINE

1.
An unstoppable growth of a university monoculture,
interested only in a narrow set of ideas
and conforming to a certain worldview,
has occurred to the detriment of open debate
and rationality.
What happened to the quest for truths?

2.
At what point do we oppose
what is wrong in modern university life?
Individuals insinuate themselves into power
by using various amalgams
of sentimentality, intimidation and false jocularity
and then wreak havoc.
Pusillanimity reigns in the academy
because protest is a disciplinary matter.

3.
Inside every rebel is a dictator trying to get out.
This is particularly true in academic medicine.

4.

Many faculty feel atomised and fearful,
waiting for the next e-mail diktat
from someone who is hard to identify
somewhere in an office,
deep in the cold-hearted control tower.

5.

The ever growing ideological and political schism
between universities and the National Health Service
is one of the causes for the malaise of academic medicine.
Both organisations must take some of the blame.

6.

Neurologists should have two
research and teaching sessions
in their NHS job plan,
and the university should actively support
clinical research by non-academics.

7.

Teaching is now the lowest of university priorities.
Research is rewarded only if it has 'impact',
a word that describes car crashes.
A radical correction is needed.

8.

Universities behave
like mediocre bureaucratic corporations.
They seem to have lost touch
with their purpose of enlightenment
at the expense of concern
with 'brand' and student satisfaction.

9.

What has happened
to the high-quality teaching
I received at medical school?
Why has imaginative experience and charisma
been discouraged
and conformity
mandated?

10.

Why are so many university academics
being pilloried by an illiberal politburo,
secreted in the inner sanctum?

11.

When I started at University College London,
the barricades and battle lines
had not yet been drawn.
We could do clinical research in the hospital,
and NHS consultants were welcomed
into the UCL academy.

12.
You write the paper, sign off copyright.
Reviewers and authors receive nothing.
Editors get a niggardly stipend.
And then the final indignity —
You need an institutional or personal subscription
to read the journal in which it is published.
Talk about rip offs!

B. ARTIFICIAL INTELLIGENCE (AI)

13.
Adoration of machines is unhealthy.
It stops humans thinking for themselves,
and even imagining.

14.
Alzheimer's dementia does not always begin
in one locus.
I am not sure we needed AI, however,
to divide it
into limbic/limbic sparing types.
Clinicians already know
that there are several recognised clinical variants.

15.
Another potential use for AI is to flag false content
and use analytics to track misinformation.
But to achieve this,
it needs to be in the hands of society,
not secretive corporations.

16.
I hope that we can use machine learning
to the benefit of our patients.
But the hard reality is that
there is no profit
in soulful neurology,
and a great deal of money
in gadgetry.

17.
There are some physicians
who love to play the numbers game
and treat the measurement,
not the patient.
Machine learning is a godsend,
and they become titans of technology,
behaving like laboratory workers.

18.
If a man aged 38
complains that the buckle of his belt
Is always to the left of centre,
and has started to lose his timing
when dancing,
what will the machine think,
and what would the zoom neurologist do?

19.

Leave machines to do the washing up,
never trust them
in matters of life and death.

20.

My concern with big data algorithms
and other AI risk predictions
is that from what I have read and seen in medicine,
they are much more likely to evolve
into curses than cures.

21.

Read any textbook description of a disease
that you are experienced in dealing with.
The discrepancy between what you read
and what you have learned
is immense.
AI could combine factual descriptions
and literature reviews,
but to what use?

22.

The term artificial intelligence
is singularly unhelpful
in understanding
what machines using algorithms
can do.

23.
There are disasters lurking behind AI diagnosis.
A brutal untreatable disease pops up
and is incorrect.
Problems getting things out of a pocket
never occurs, for example,
as a first symptom
in Richardson's syndrome[1].

24.
Those of you who value democracy and altruism,
stay clear of machine learning.
Even if it can be controlled by citizens,
which I doubt,
it will destroy scholarship
and become an instrument
of malign oligarchy.

25.
Scholars, Craftsmen, Artists,
resist AI
wherever and whenever
you have the chance.

---

[1] Richardson's syndrome is a neurodegenerative disorder also known as Progressive Supranuclear Palsy-RS characterised by an inability to move the eyes up and down, unexplained falls backwards, a growling speech and slowed movements with the abnormal accumulation of abnormal tau protein in the brain. It is named after J. Clifford Richardson (1909-1986), a Toronto neurologist.

26.

We must humanise machine learning
and medical technology
before it dehumanises us.

27.

What is the neurological cause
for a self-winding Rolex watch
stopping repeatedly
despite regular servicing?
Run the question through ChatGPT[2]
and if it comes up with the answer,
we can be certain
that our pockets have been picked.

28.

What will the AI algorithm come up with
when a 64-year-old businessman complains
that he can't put his hand
in his trouser pocket,
and thinks there is a design fault
in his suit?
Only one diagnosis likely here,
and it's Parkinson's disease.

---

[2] ChatGPT is a generative artificial intelligence chatbot that uses
large language models.

29.
I am opposed
to the algorithmic approach
to medicine.
It is profligate and dangerous.
What we need
are more well-trained physicians and surgeons,
a simple and dependable solution
that will also save money
in the long run.

C. Art

30.
Marvelous van Gogh inundation virtual reality exhibition
at 106 Commercial Street in the East End,
evidence that his brilliant colours
stemmed from Daltonism.
Cypresses, Sunflowers, Starry skies,
Crows and Dr Gachet[3].

31.
Sitting on a deck chair
in the old stable building
across the road from Spitalfields,
thinking of the unbearable mental agony
that accompanied van Gogh's painting.
Immersed for an hour
in a landscape
created by memory
as well as observation.

---

[3] *The portrait of Dr Gachet* is one of Vincent van Gogh's most celebrated paintings. Paul Gachet was an artist and doctor who took care of van Gogh in the last months of his life.

32.

Dance your Parkinson's away,
from early morning until late at night.
You fill my heart with pure delight,
Dopamine release.

33.

Everything that had puzzled me was clear.
Why I had fallen under the spell of Motown[4].
How 'the D'[5] had saved my soul
in the darkest of days.
The fascinating paradox of Henry Ford[6].

34.

I give money to St Mungo's[7] and the Sally Army[8]
by direct debit.
On the street I never give to beggars
with sad dogs sitting on carpets,
but always to Balkan accordion players,
who raise my spirit
with their tunes.

---

[4] Motown Records was an influential record label founded in 1959 by Berry Gordy Jr. in Detroit.
[5] The 'D' is a nickname for Detroit.
[6] Henry Ford (1863-1947), American industrialist who made automobiles affordable for ordinary Americans through a system that became known as Fordism.
[7] St Mungo's is a charity to help people experiencing homelessness.
[8] The Salvation Army is a Protestant Christian church and an international charitable organisation.
[9] A novel written by William Seward Burroughs in 1959.

35.

After I had read *Naked Lunch*[9],
I tried to develop rigorous methodologies
of self-knowledge
that would assist neurological phenomenology.

36.

During his life,
William Burroughs[10] became more and more concerned
with the destruction of the earth
and the boundless power of oligarchs.
Everything he scryed is true,
and now nothing is permitted.
Take a moment to read his prescient piece
from Nova Express[11].

37.

Diderot showed us
that the novel is defined
by a timeless uncertainty,
which is why reading books
helps physicians
in the diagnostic process,
and their attendance.

---

[10] William Seward Burroughs (1914-1997) was an American post-modernist writer and visual artist.
[11] A 1964 novel by William Burroughs written using the fold-in method, a version of the cut-up developed with Brion Gysin.

38.

I read *Jude the Obscure*
when I was uncertain
about my future in medicine.
I have read *Tess of the d'Urbervilles* now,
at the backend of my career.
Both make me sob.
It is not about injustice alone.

39.

Hardy[12] takes me to places
that I have never reached
through reading Dickens.

40.

This morning my mind
is full of archipelagos.
But then I think of the richness
of John Clare's[13] life,
where he felt no need
to travel beyond the horizon.
He knew there was nothing better
in Peterborough, London or Northampton.
Helpston was where he belonged.

---

[12] Thomas Hardy (1840-1928), English novelist and poet, author of
Jude the Obscure and *Tess of the d'Urbervilles*.
[13] John Clare (1793-1864), an English nature poet.

41.

You need to read A.J. Cronin's[14] book
The Citadel
to understand why Doyle's[15] ophthalmological practice
failed miserably
on Upper Wimpole Street.
His rather bluff demeanour
probably didn't help either.

42.

J.G. Ballard[16] studied medicine at Kings Cambridge
for two years
from 1949-51.
But he gave up
because he felt
all the factual learning required
was damaging his imagination.
He left without a degree
and a mild disappointment
that he could not become
a psychiatrist.

---

[14] A.J. Cronin (1896-1981), a Scottish physician and novelist.
[15] Arthur Conan Doyle (1859-1930), British writer and physician.
[16] J.G. Ballard (1930-2009), English novelist, short story writer who did two years of study in medicine.

D. Bad Medicine

43.

Galenical physicians
trained at universities
prefer not to touch patients.
All they do
is gaze at a screen.

44.

Dumbing down
or settling for a second-rate option
should be anathema
in life
and in medicine.

45.

I am often sent a pile of test results
to comment on:
Neurophysiology, imaging, genetic and metabolic screens,
but no accompanying neurologist's letter
documenting the medical history,
the examination findings,
or the clinical opinion.

46.

Keep androids
out of clinical medicine.
They can be recognised
by their gauche and risible clinical skills,
by their absence of empathy and compassion,
by their large but unstructured knowledge base,
and by their heavy reliance
on technology of questionable accuracy.
We all know them.

47.

Androids are very fond
of arcane and elitist abbreviations
and of acronyms
which patients do not understand.
They also adore words
like dysdiadochokinesia[17]
And dysmetria[18].

---

[17] Dysdiadochokinesia is difficulty in performing rapid alternating movements due to dysfunction of the cerebellum (hind brain).
[18] Dysmetria is difficulty in judging the distance, speed and range of motion needed for coordinated movement and is often caused by damage to the cerebellum (hind brain).

48.

I do not 'deliver care',
another egregious term like health provider,
designed to create barriers
between physician and patient
and diminish the art of healing.

49.

I do not want to work as a doctor
or live in a country
where expensive unnecessary investigations are available,
but there are no ophthalmoscopes,
peak flow meters,
or urine dip sticks.

50.

Nor do I wish to practice
in a place where there are many highly trained specialists
for the rich
but no connected referral pathways.

51.

I grow tired of being manipulated
by basic scientists and medical academics
who rarely see patients
but who are imbued with righteous certainty
and try to influence clinical practice.

52.

I grow tired of the expanding business
of disease mongering
and the branding of spurious syndromes
for profit.

53.

I saw a patient
whose last neurologist
started glancing at his watch
after about 15 minutes
and who asked not a single question
about her life.

54.
It is illogical
to reduce a patient's symptoms and signs
to fixed emanations.
In an instant,
tremor 3 becomes tremor 0,
making the point score meaningless,
nothing more than a momentary reaction
to a particular stimulus.

55.
Most physicians see
only what they are looking for
and recognise as significant
only what they know.
Medicine is difficult,
and a closed mind
makes it harder.

56.
My seven modern medical sins are:
Indifference
Technophilia
Passivity
Hubris
Customer friendliness
Hype
and Hyposkillia.

57.
The measurement
has become both the malady
and the outcome.
Clinimetrics taken to extreme is a form of medicine
where a panel of tests is ordered
for machines to do
and someone else to interpret.

58.
Scans ordered without thought
are not a harmless extravagance.
They may create ephemeral reassurance,
or more likely unnecessary distress,
especially for the asymptomatic
and those anxious about their health.

59.

See your physician if you are ill.
Don't let profiteering overdiagnosis
and disease mongering
get a grip on you.

60.

I am concerned
about my speciality of Movement Disorders.
Its current obsession
with meaningless measures,
premature biological definitions,
Spanophilia[19],
and synuclein aggregation
have created
an increasingly barren field.

---

[19] Spanophilia is an excessive love of rare, exotic and obscure syndromes.

61.

When medical experts
propose a new syndrome,
especially when there are no pathognomonic signs,
be on your guard.
The media and medical industrial complex
usually then get involved,
and before you can blink,
a nebulous malady is born
that enters the vernacular
and starts to be worn by victims
as a badge of honour.

62.

We used to have a 4-point scale in therapeutics
relating to overall improvement —
None, slight, moderate and marked.
To describe the improvement with lecanemab[20]
as 'moderate'
is deceitful.

---

[20] Lecanemab is an antibody directed against amyloid and
administered intravenously which has been licensed for the
treatment of Alzheimer's disease despite having negligible benefit
and serious side effects.

63.

As the sky darkens,
and as storm clouds gather,
there is a light,
even though it may be seen only rarely
and in occasional faint glimpses.
This is how I feel
about progress in neurology.
Yet there are complacent colleagues
who walk around
as if they are bathed in sunlight.

64.

When someone with Parkinson's disease
starts on levodopa[21],
the improvement is usually striking
to patient, family and doctor.
I wonder how neurologists
who prescribe lecanemab
are evaluating its effectiveness,
as deterioration continues?

---

[21] Levodopa is a naturally occurring amino acid precursor of the chemical messenger dopamine used to treat Parkinson's disease.

65.

My fear is that,
like the use of dopamine transporter scans[22]
for the investigation
of possible Parkinson's disease,
the blood test for amyloid
will be used by doctors,
who should be working in laboratories
as a surrogate,
for careful longitudinal clinical evaluation.

66.

The biological approach to Alzheimer's[23]
has led to chaos.

67.

Having good intentions
doesn't make you a good doctor
or a healer.

---

[22] Dopamine transporter scans (DAT) is a test based on single
photon emission tomography used to measure dopamine uptake in
the brain. In Parkinson's disease, reduction in transporter uptake is
seen in the basement of the brain.
[23] Alzheimer's disease is now used by some clinicians for mild
cognitive impairment but no dementia.

68.

Goodhart's Law[24]:
'When a measure becomes a target,
it ceases to be a good measure.'

69.

I find it disturbing
that some colleagues
have rigid algorithmic prescribing habits.
They have a limited feel
for the action of molecules
and what each can do.
They don't see much purpose
in adjusting their recommendations
to a patient's life or wishes.
A pharmacist can do that.

---

[24] Goodhart's Law warns that once the focus shifts from achieving the desired outcome to simply achieving the target itself then catastrophe is never far away.

E. Deep Medicine

70.

I have found that the academics
who talk about personalised medicine
never mention individual people.
Only big data, artificial intelligence,
and algorithms.
I wish they would accept
that what they are promoting
is impersonal and inhuman.

71.

'Deep biology approach to Alzheimer's disease'.
The latest garbage hyperbole
joins the demeaning deep medicine
and deep phenotyping.
If you hear these terms,
be instantly sceptical.
They are Peacockian
and slyly try to denigrate
good clinical practice.

72.
There is a lot of chatter
about 'precision medicine'.
But I have yet to read
an exact and clear explanation
of how it differs
from best medical practice.

73.
'Deep medicine'
needs to be left
to drown in the shallows.
It is condescending
and inappropriate.
Those who seem fond of the notion
also seem incapable
of using precise prose
to define its distinctive characteristics.

F. Elevated Practice

74.
Always strive
for exactness and keenness
in observation.
And then analyse
the cognitive processes
by which each fact is deduced,
remembering that it is always more complicated
than it first appears.

75.
As a doctor,
one encounters the tenderest
and most vulnerable parts
of human nature.
Physicians need to understand
the modes of thought and feelings
of the sick
and always treat them
with gentleness.

76.
Being a physician
has never been a burden for me.
It is an honour
and a privilege
far greater than being asked to give a plenary speech.

77.
Enthusiasm is the key
to leadership and success
in medicine.
You cannot fake it.

78.
Chat with the experts.
Make new connections.
Think about how what you heard
might improve your clinical practice.
And ask the question,
'Is this something
that could help my patients now?'

79.

I have never seen neurology
as a job.
I have never felt
I didn't want to go into work.
If you lose your enthusiasm
or imagine yourself in another job,
then you become a menace
and must retire immediately.

80.

If I am in doubt,
I want to be able
to refer to a colleague
who meticulously records her opinion
in the notes.

81.

I want to work in a place
where I have a responsibility
for my patients,
where there is minimal wastage
of resources,
and where overdiagnosis
Is frowned upon.

82.
It is not enough
to pleasantly follow guidelines
and clock off.
There are occasions
when you need
to break convention.

83.
Neurology is subjective.
In addition to observation and listening,
other valuable attributes
for a practitioner
are intuition, compassion, and urbanity.
And common sense.

84.
Nothing now gives me greater pleasure
than seeing my students and fellows
outstrip me in every way.
It is my negligible contribution
to the advancement of civilisation.

85.

To be a neurologist,
you need to be a good doctor,
an enthusiastic teacher,
and a clinical researcher.
All 3 are possible
but nowadays
harder to achieve.

86.

Question dogma.
Remain sceptical.
Double check your sources of information.
And make the clinic your laboratory.

87.

To make patients better,
you don't necessarily need
to prescribe medication,
to operate,
or even to make a firm diagnosis.
But you do need
to give realistic hope,
to show compassion and understanding,
and be thorough in your approach.

88.
Question everything,
but do not doubt everything.
Always search for the truth
in your daily practice.

89.
Your white coat
is a symbol of compassion.
A beacon of hope.
A shield against suffering.
It is a conduit
through which flow
empathy and understanding.
Your coat is the weight
and privilege
you carry as a physician
and the weight of the lives
of the people you touch.

90.

Medicine is not a bullshit job.
For most of us, nor
is it a calling like the priesthood.
I see it as a practical art
that requires sound judgement
and tacit knowledge
for its best practice.
It is a grown-up craft.

91.

Before giving a diagnosis,
I need to know
about the domestic situation.
The family.
The patient's occupation.
These are not optional extras.
They shape how one explains
changes that will happen with the disease.

G. Etiquette

92.
Disregard and indifference to dress
is a sign of egotism.
Not a sign of a free spirit
or of a mind fixed on higher things.

93.
If you know more than someone
about a subject
and dare to express it,
you are at risk
of being branded a pedant
or a nerd.
If you know less
or just elect to remain silent,
you may be branded dim
or ignorant.

94.
People, people!
If you want to find a good neurologist,
never consult
any name that pops up
when you google,
'The top neurologists'.
It is an even more perilous method of inquiry
if you replace 'neurologist'
with 'Parkinson's disease specialist'.

95.
Self-deprecation
is a protection
against criticism.
The English excel in it.
Self-righteousness
is an emotion
that never disappoints,
and one which can last
a lifetime.

96.
The doctors I respect
have no time
for social media platforms
or self-promotion
on glossy websites.
'Personal branding'
is an expression
of one's soul
through one's vocation.
A good reputation comes
by selfless application.

97.
The neurologist I want to see
when I get sick
needs to be a generalist
with a specialist eye.
A humanist
with a touch of the supernatural.
And a physician
who finds as much interest
In Bell's Palsy[25]
as in hereditary congenital facial paralysis.
Scientism is not essential.

---

[25] Bell's Palsy is a common sudden weakness usually of one side of the face and which usually recovers spontaneously in a few weeks. Its cause is unknown.

H. Exotic Disorders

98.

A genetic disease
presenting in middle age
with unsteadiness and oscillopsia[26],
with sensory symptoms and a cough.
And examination reveals
impaired vestibular ocular reflexes[27]
and a neuropathy.
It has an acronym,
but at least a memorable one,
reminding us of a durable fabric
used to make tents[28].

---

[26] Oscillopsia is a visual disturbance in which objects in the visual field move or jump.

[27] Vestibular ocular reflex is a reflex that stabilises vision by producing eye movements that counteract movements of the head and neck.

[28] CANVAS syndrome is a rare genetic neurological disorder in adults characterised by unsteadiness, loss of power and sensation in the limbs due to a peripheral nerve disturbance (neuropathy) and loss of balance and eye movement control.

99.

A genetic disorder
presenting with pyramidal weakness[29],
with severe dysarthria[30]
and with frontal signs.
It is not C9orf72[31],
which I have finally committed to memory:
Orfe is a fish,
And 72 was my Paris year.
It is TBK1,
a TANK kinase mutation[32].
What's in a name?
A great deal of money!

---

[29] Pyramidal weakness is loss of power in the limbs due to damage to the nervous pathways in the central nervous system.
[30] Dysarthria is a disorder of speech articulation.
[31] C9Orf72 is the commonest genetic cause of motor neurone disease (amyotrophic lateral sclerosis).
[32] A TANK-binding kinase (TBK1) mutation refers to a change in the DNA sequence leading to altered protein function and linked to amyotrophic lateral sclerosis and frontotemporal dementia.

100.

Does anyone know
which fool proposed the eponym
Diogenes syndrome[33]
for pathological hoarding?
I love eponyms in modest dosage.
But this is one of the least appropriate
in the literature.

101.

A rare genetic disease of adolescents,
first reported from the village
of Kufor Rakeb
in Jordan.
It presents with L-DOPA responsive bradykinesia[34]
with supranuclear gaze palsy[35]
with myoclonus of the chin,
and with dystonia[36].
We know the gene too,
even if its name
is hard to recall!

---

[33] Diogenes syndrome is a disorder characterised by extreme self-neglect, domestic squalor, hoarding of rubbage or animals and social withdrawal.
[34] Bradykinesia is a progressive reduction in the speed and amplitude of repetitive voluntary movement and is a sine qua non for the diagnosis of Parkinson's disease.
[35] Supranuclear gaze palsy is an inability to look in a particular direction which often gives the eyes a staring appearance. It is a characteristic feature of Richardson's syndrome (PSP).
[36] Dystonia is an abnormal posturing leading to contortions.

I. FOOTBALL

102.
Bill Shankly[37]
was another great influence
on my career,
along with my neurological teachers
and the scrying of William Burroughs.
No wonder 'Shank's' players
would give everything
in every game.
No Liverpool manager
has come close since.

---

[37] Bill Shankly 'Shanks' (1913-1981) was a Scottish football player
best remembered for his time as manager of Liverpool Football
Club (1959-1974).

103.

Does anyone else turn off
the football commentary on television?
The lack of excitement,
the Gradgrindian meaningless statistics,
the television referee
commenting on the referee,
the VAR delays[38].
I want Spanish or Brazilian commentators
who are free
to express passion.

104.

Football has glorious moments
always unrelated
to the game's result.
But it can never reach
the utter ineffability and soulfulness
of JJ Barnes[39]
or of Levi Stubbs[40]
belting out a banger.
But both can kick out Parkinson's.

---

[38] VAR (video assistant referee) is a football match official who assists the referee with the help of film footage and other technologies.
[39] JJ Barnes (1943-2022) was an American singer and songwriter who became very popular on the Northern Soul circuit.
[40] Levi Stubbs (1936-2008) was lead singer of the Four Tops Detroit group who had numerous hit records, initially with Motown records and then on other labels.

J. LANGUAGE

105.
A neurologist
is neither a health care provider
nor a brain surgeon,
not even a 'neuro'.
A neurologist is a physician.

106.
A patient is a citizen.
A patient is not a client or a consumer
or even a sufferer.
Words matter.

107.
In Medicine,
we need to be ever more alert
to language
that bewitches thought.

108.

Can anyone tell me
what a keynote speech is?
I know it will be long
and delivered by a high-profile person
who wields power,
but is it ever truly a central theme?

109.

An eminent Spanish colleague
and a polyglot
told me that
he had some difficulty
understanding British speakers
at international neurology conferences.
The problem was partly due to accent
but also to the use of words
and to the grammar and prosody.
The language differed
from scientific lingua franca.

110.

I prefer eponymous lectures
like the Oslerian Oration[41],
because the audience
get a couple of history slides,
and the speaker a medal,
rather than an honorarium.

111.

'Hospitalise' is another dehumanising word
that should be avoided.
Hospitals are complex ecosystems,
not impersonal assembly lines.
Try instead 'Mr Smith
was admitted to the hospital'.

112.

The best tweets can express much
in very few words.
It was that possibility and constraint
that first drew me to Twitter.

---

[41] William Osler (1849-1919) was a Canadian physician frequently
described as the Father of Modern Medicine because of his
consummate clinical method.

113.
I am weary of hurrah words
like 'progressive'
and 'state of the art'.
Like 'innovative'
and 'game-changing'.
And of boo words
like 'outdated'
and 'wasteful'.
Like 'last century'
and 'traditional'.

114.
I dislike euphemisms
in everyday speech.
But they are very valuable in medicine,
provided they are not falsehoods.

115.
You should smell a rat
if a medical scientist,
when presenting at conferences
or in a publication,
does not use
straightforward plain language.

116.

In England we are judged
not only by our accents
but by every single word we use.
Appearance is a secondary factor.

117.

Lucidity and brevity
are the soul of style.
Never use two words
where one will do.

118.

The common language we share
is not about rules
but about effective communication.
And about intelligibility.

119.

The spoken and the written word
should be beautiful and inspiring.
I'm always working
to get better at both.

K. THE MEDIA

120.

Over the years,
I have found
the Today programme
on BBC Radio 4
to be the best national media outlet
to get a feel for the impact
of a new scientific finding.
The broadsheets are now
as bad as the tabloids.

121.

Why do journalists always say
someone is 'fighting for their life'
when it has been announced
that the person is comatose
and being kept alive
by assisted ventilation?

122.

Why do the weather ladies always talk
of the promise of sunshine
and the threat of rain?
Why can't they be more specific
about the type of expected rain?
And I don't mean showers or drizzle,
I mean the feel of the rain
on my face.

123.

It pleases me
to see more people
on the Tube
reading books with covers.
There are very few using tablets.
But the smart phone
still rules the roost.

124.

To see anyone reading a national newspaper
on the Tube
is a rarity.
Even free copy
like *Metro* and *Standard*
is much less in evidence.

L. MEDICINE AND POLITICS

125.

The continuing attempts
by NHS England
and by Hospital Trusts
to destroy case notes
will cost lives and money,
and will be another nail in the coffin
for clinical research.

126.

A lot of waffle
about the importance
of NHS data
and the need to do better
in primary care.
But we know the truth.
The shredding and rubbing out goes on
without consultation.

127.

Despite their remoteness from reality,
some academic eminences try to control
how neurology is practised.

128.
I do not want to work in a system
dictated to by deceitful 'not for profit' health providers
and by greedy medical insurance firms.

129.
I am thinking today
of the patients and staff
in the emergency room
of the Royal Liverpool Hospital.
Money must be found
for front line care,
to repair the immense harm
done by the last government,
to improve working conditions,
and to give hope.
No more inquiries!

130.
I hope the new Labour government
will talk less
about 'modernising'
the 'broken' NHS
and more
about restoring quality of care.
And about improving morale
through improved working conditions.

131.

I saw the best neurologists of my generation
demoralised by red tape
and by tabloid newspapers,
their craft denigrated
by government.
By insurance companies.
By bean counters.
By electronic health records.
By low touch telemedicine.
By the Royal College of Physicians.
and by the GMC.

132.

I'm keen on watchful waiting in medicine
but not in politics.

133.

I want to see a government
that has an immediate
and a futuristic perspective
to world problems.
William Burroughs was right,
'We are running out of time'.

134.

I am opposed
to short term individualism
and to rule
by technocrats.

135.

If you had symptoms,
would you want to be seen
by the chairman of neurology
at an Ivy league university?
Or by a neurologist
who likes people
and has a general competence?

136.

People, people!
Choose your general practitioner with care,
and if you get on well
and have trust and faith,
stick with her.

137.

Avoid profiteers
bearing false promises
who deride, erode and parasitise
the NHS[42].
Remember the glossy emporia,
always cry for help
when the going gets tough,
or when your insurance pot
runs dry.

---

[42] NHS is the National Health Service, the publicly funded healthcare system of the United Kingdom established in 1948 with the principle of being universal, comprehensive and free at the point of delivery.

138.

The reduced interest
in vocational training
to become a doctor
has more to do with NHS working conditions
than with pay.
It has a little bit to do too
with best-selling books
written by disillusioned doctors.

139.

This shambolic Tory government[43]
has no interest
in the continuing shortage
of efficacious medications.
Instead,
it backs new, expensive me-too placebos
and sweeteners,
urged on by the powerful medical charities.

---

[43] A tweet inspired by the Conservative government's inability to draw attention to the negligible value of the new anti-amyloid drugs for people living with Alzheimer's disease and their muddled dementia awareness initiative.

140.

Jargon-ridden terms
coming out of the health insurance board rooms
and out of the NHS control tower
have contaminated our hospitals
Like superbugs.
They are at best piffle
and at worst viruses
that attack the sanctity
of the medical consultation.

141.

Still a platform soul.
I am hoping
that nationalisation of the railways,
as well as the water companies,
is on the cards
once the NHS
is fully restored.

142.

Private health companies
should not be allowed to advertise,
claiming to be 'not for profit'
because it is mendacious.
For a start,
look at the salaries
of their CEOs[44].

---

[44] CEO is an abbreviation for Chief Executive Officer.

M. NATURE

143.
Amazonia is now
the centre of human consciousness.
We must reforest our minds
and engage.
Donate if you can
to WWF.
To Survival International.
To Rainforest Trust.

144.
During lockdown,
I did some field work
on the garden robin.
It took me until the next Spring
to discover it was a hen robin.
The robin is a bird
with fascinating behaviour
and a deceiving appearance.

145.
Global warning has turned English weather
into dull climate.
A topic of interest
only for meteorologists
and hypochondriacs.
The once eagerly anticipated vagaries
has changed into stuck-in set isobars.

146.
I'm talking about pelting rain.
Lashing rain.
Cold rain.
Mizzle.
Misty rain.
Damp rain.
Gentle rain.
Soaking, tepid rain.

147.

Snow is so infrequent now
in the South of England
that I have come to look on snowfall
as a magical event,
decorated by its stealthiness and silence.
Waking to a white glistening level
is like being on board ship.
I am sick for now
of grey featureless days of rain,
and of raw wind.

148.

The dawn symphony intensifies
as the days lengthen.
In Cherry Tree Woods[45]
I heard great and blue tits.
Wrens and robins.
A song thrush, a crow and a magpie.
And an early blackcap.
My ear now hears
what my eyes cannot see.
Listening with intent.

---

[45] Cherry Tree Woods is a small, picturesque park in East Finchley
which has become an enclave for nature.

149.
Yesterday at the feeding station,
there were 6 carrion crows,
2 jackdaws,
and 4 magpies.
Today only the wood pigeons turned up,
weather unchanged.
I'll turn to ornithomancy
to work it out.
The mystery of the birds.

N. Neurological Skills

150.
In neurology,
as for detective work,
you learn early on
that often the best way
to solve a diagnostic problem
is neither the quickest
nor the least interesting.
The history,
then a focused examination.
Selected tests if necessary.
And finally,
tacit knowledge.

151.

I encourage neurologists
to use their ears
not only for attentive listening
to the history,
but also for cranial bruits[46]
and helicopter signs[47].
And the most neglected of all,
'the sound of footsteps',
which can be diagnostic.

152.

An excellent strong response
to a first dose of 25/100 mg levodopa
does not point
to functional Parkinson's syndrome,
but an instantaneous one does.
What a difference
an hour makes.

---

[46] Bruit is a whooshing or swishing sound heard with a stethoscope
when listening over an artery and which may be of pathological
significance.
[47] Helicopter sign is a high frequency sound resembling a distant
helicopter heard by listening with a stethoscope over the thigh
muscle and when present may indicate a nervous disorder called
orthostatic tremor.

153.

When I started out

in neurology,

accurate diagnosis,

was the be all,

and almost the end all.

Magnetic resonance imaging

and other tests

have made this step

a little easier.

But in neurology,

it is still challenging.

Once it is secure,

the next step involves

soulful neurology[48].

Do you know what I'm talking about?

---

[48] Soulful Neurology is a method of neurological practice which does not diminish patients to crude measurements, their diagnostic label or their treatment regimen. It requires a holistic approach that depends on a punctilious clinical method but also embraces the mystery and magic of life. I coined the term in my book *Brainspotting: Adventures in Neurology,* where I drew a distinction between it and psychiatry.

154.

Inspection as a useful diagnostic method
gradually reduced in importance
as the neurological examination
became more developed
in the early 20th century.

155.

Go out and get that story.
You will never get anywhere
sitting on your dead tail.
Not just any story.
Not just any picture.
But *the clinical story*.
And *the clinical picture*.
This is the business
of neurology.

156.

I always ask people
where they grew up,
as well as what they do
for a living,
because it occasionally gives
diagnostic clues.
It also has some effect
on a person's virtues
and humours.

157.

I have never done this,
but there are one or two colleagues,
and not only those,
with a training in genetics
who start the medical interview
with the family history.

158.

In straightforward cases,
a brief and simple interrogation
is often adequate.
In difficult cases,
time spent in going deeper
into the clinical history
is never time wasted.

159.

When taking a history,
never ask the same question twice.
And when listening
to a patient's story,
never look surprised.
Or perplexed.

160.
What happens to a 32-year-old woman
who complains of a cold white left hand
and a painful shoulder
who doesn't get to see a physician
face-to-face?
If she is fortunate,
she will see a physiotherapist
who will correctly diagnose Parkinson's
and arrange a referral.

161.
What would happen to a 59-year-old man
whose first symptom
is that when driving,
he involuntarily veers slightly
to the middle of the road?
Will he be subjected
to 'on referral' algorithmic medicine?
This is an early visuospatial difficulty
that occasionally is the first symptom
of Parkinsons disease.

162.

I have seen several patients
who presented with pulsatile tinnitus.
A structural vascular cause
was never found.
Instead of emphasising glomus tumours,
carotid stenosis and dural A-V fistulas
as likely causes in the neurological texts,
conductive hearing loss needs to be given more emphasis,
as it is far commoner.

O. Neurological Pearls

163.
Copper rings,
blue moons,
and sunflowers.
A disease called Wilson[49].

164.
If you have night starvation,
take Horlicks.
If you have daily fatigue,
take Feroglobin.
If you are over 65
and can't remember a name,
have your amyloid test?
Poppycock!

---

[49] Wilson's disease is a rare genetic disorder which leads to copper accumulation in the body and presents most often in childhood and adolescence with cirrhosis, abnormal movements and neuropsychiatric symptoms, green-brown discolouration of the cornea, sunflower cataracts and azure discolouration of the white part of the nails.

165.

Understanding
is usually the best way
to relieve a medical problem.

166.

Neurologists are a necessary evil,
just like the police.
They should behave like good coppers on the beat,
constantly on the alert,
always noticing.
And when mischief occurs,
deal with it efficiently and innocuously.

167.

Charisma, confidence,
and the use of silent language
are teaching gifts
that should be encouraged.
All are instantly blunted
by telemedicine.

168.

Only observation is certain.
The transition between theory and fact is gradual.
And much of what neurologists believe
is subjective.

169.
Always surround yourself
with young people
smarter and cleverer than yourself.
And allow them to fly free.

170.
Question everything,
but do not doubt everything.
Always search for the truth
in your daily practice.

171.
My few original thoughts have come
when I am walking or reading
or lying in bed.
Never in front of a blank page.
This is why I always have a notebook
and pencil to hand.

172.
Molecular genetics hurtles ahead
with new gene errors found daily.
I find it hard to remember
most of the mutations,
especially when they describe proteins.

173.

The SCA[50] and PARK[51] schemes
are unmanageable
for the average medical brain.

174.

This morning,
I am fighting a fear
that originality is no longer possible
and that I am no more
than a programmed computer.

175.

Those fears,
that despite our little idiosyncrasies
we are all mass produced
in the same genetic factory,
have recurred.
If correct,
they preclude any chance
of seeking a better world
in Brazil.

---

[50] SCA is an abbreviation for spinocerebellar atrophy, a disorder
which has many causes including 40 genetic disorders. The
classification gives each identified mutation a number, e.g. SCA3.
[51] PARK is an abbreviation for Parkinsonism with numbers
similarly being used to distinguish the different genetic forms, e.g.
PARK 1.

176.
Advice for Parkinson's disease specialists:
learn from colleagues
at the forefront of diabetes research.
Restore academic clinical neuropharmacology.
And consider new work
on dopamine.

177.
Neurologists should ponder questions
asked by patients in clinic
to which the only honest answer
is 'I don't know'.
If after careful consideration
and a detailed literature review
back to 1860,
'Not known' is the answer,
then you have a research project.

178.

Guidelines and recommendations
only have value
if the tensions and assumptions
emerging during their development
are revealed,
then vigorously debated,
by doctors and patients.
This never happens.
So they end up at best
a crude start to effective care,
not an end.

179.

I prefer to think of illness
in terms of suffering,
not as a measurement
that purports to demarcate
health from disease.

180.
The London Hospital, Whitechapel,
put neurological paraneoplastic syndromes[52]
on the map.
The papers from Brain, Croft and Henson[53]
were greeted with scepticism
at Queen Square[54],
where few cancer patients,
brain tumours apart,
were seen.
Just because you haven't seen it
doesn't mean it doesn't exist.

---

[52] Paraneoplastic syndromes are a group of conditions causing symptoms that are not explained by the primary cancer or its metastatic spread, which are due to chemical substances produced by the tumour or by an immune response to the tumour.
[53] Russel Brain, Peter Croft and Ronald Henson were three neurologists working at the London Hospital in the early 1960s.
[54] Queen Square is sometimes used to refer to the National Hospital for Neurology and Neurosurgery in London.

181.

'Brain fog[55]

and the more recent and distinct 'Brain rot[56]

are terms that have been promulgated

through lay use,

mainly on social media.

Like 'catarrh' and 'indigestion',

they need breaking down

into the different subjective phenomena

experienced in each case.

182.

Mild memory impairment,

difficulties in expression,

mental dullness,

and muzziness.

These form a cluster of symptoms

that are commonly reported

by people with Parkinson's disease.

And they are usually intermittent.

Is this brain fog?

My patients rarely use that term

in their description.

---

[55] Brain fog describes a cloudy fuzzy feeling in the head making it hard to concentrate.

[56] Brain rot is a term used to describe a perceived mental decline due to excessive consumption of trivial online social media content.

183.

In people with Parkinson's disease,
I have tended to link occasional 'senior moments'
and 'mental blocks',
groggy feelings and depersonalisation,
more with 'off period' depression
than with cognitive decline.

184.

Remember
that patients with many symptoms
are always at greater risk
of receiving multiple diagnoses.
And some of these labels will be nebulous
and even erroneous.

185.

The problem with Linnaean[57] taxonomy for physicians
is that molecular genetics
has created a very different nosology,
which transcends external appearance
and even histopathology.

---

[57] Carl Linnaeus (1707-1778) was a Swedish biologist and physician who formalised the binomial nomenclature classification for all living things.

186.

Thomas Sydenham[58] said
'It is necessary
that all diseases be reduced
to definite and certain species
and that, with the same care we see shown
by botanists in their phytologies.
He would be a careless botanist indeed
who only exhibited the marks
by which the class was identified'.

---

[58] Thomas Sydenham (1624-1689) was a physician who wrote a textbook of medicine and became known as the English Hippocrates.

187.
Do psychiatrists take any interest
in Burton's[59] 'windy melancholy'?
Wind rumbles,
belly-ache,
heat in the bowels?
Convulsive spasms,
crudities,
and sour and sharp belchings?
The best medical treatment
is a psychotropic –
low dose amitriptyline[60].
I still like and use
the unfashionable term
psychosomatic.

---

[59] Robert Burton, a scholar who wrote a medical treatise and pathography called *The Anatomy of Melancholy* in 1621.
[60] Amitriptyline hydrochloride is a psychotropic medication that prolongs the activity of serotonin and noradrenaline in the brain and relieves depression, pain, some forms of headache and irritable bowel syndrome.

P. NORTHERN SOUL

188.
Northern Soul
is about unknowability.
It is also about
brilliant dance music.
Its best disc jockeys
have a good ear for floor fillers,
and in a way become surrogate A and R men,
but they are not high priests.

189.
Finsbury Park, Hornsey,
Alexandra Palace, Oakleigh Park,
New Barnet, Hadley Wood,
Potters Bar, Brookmans Park.
Welham Green and Hatfield coach stations
on the spinal East Coast Line,
running parallel
to the Great and Old North Roads.
Walk on.
A new beginning.
Northern soul.

190.
The origin of the moves in Northern Soul
is obscure.
But probably Bruce Lee
is not a major contributor.
And the Mills Brothers, Jackie Wilson and James Brown,
may be less influential than once thought.
The can-can, for example,
has kicks, splits and somersaults.

191.
Is Northern Soul
the only thriving dance movement
in the UK?
Up and down the land,
clubs and dance halls are closing.
Health-conscious millennials
are staying home.
You don't need alcohol or white powder
to get high
when Edwin Starr[61] and Major Lance[62]
are on the decks.

---

[61] Edwin Starr (1942-2003) was an American singer who became the most influential and popular artist on the British Northern soul scene in the 1970s.
[62] Major Lance (1939-1994) was an American R&B singer who became a cult figure on the Northern Soul scene.

Q. Nostalgia

192.
I was a pupil
until I went to medical college,
then I became a student.
I rarely hear the word pupil now,
even at my grandchildren's primary school.

193.

It is a tragedy
that the teaching autopsy has disappeared
and that brain banking,
to which the MRC[63] pays lip service,
has had to rely for 20 years
on charitable support.
In neurodegeneration[64] and stroke,
in multiple sclerosis[65] and 'organic' psychiatry,
the post-mortem is the final diagnostic service
offered to the patient.
In neurodegeneration[66] and stroke,
in multiple sclerosis and 'organic' psychiatry,
the post-mortem is the final diagnostic service
offered to the patient.

---

[63] MRC: abbreviation of Medical Research Council which is the United Kingdom funding agency dedicated to improving human health by supporting research.
[64] Neurodegenerative disease includes common conditions like Alzheimer's disease and Parkinson's disease characterised by focal loss of nerve cells in the brain, the cause of which remains obscure.
[65] Multiple sclerosis is an adult-onset immunological disturbance of the central nervous system which damages the myelin insulation covers of nerve cells. It can relapse and remit over years or less commonly be relentlessly progressive.
[66] Neurodegenerative disease includes common conditions like Alzheimer's disease and Parkinson's disease characterised by focal loss of nerve cells in the brain, the cause of which remains obscure.

194.
We all wanted to die young.
We didn't want to look or be like our parents,
even when we loved them.
We had money to burn.
The oral contraceptive
promised limitless possibility.
National Service had been abolished,
and there were the new discotheques.

195.
When doctors met regularly
in a common room,
perplexing symptoms
spanning specialities
were discussed.
Cross referrals were seamless.
Now it is an electronic referral
without soul or nuance.

196.
Like the Aymara[67],
the future is always behind me
and unforeseeable.
While the past is there
in front of my eyes.
I walk forwards,
on the march to oblivion,
facing an Elysian past.

197.
We visited South Ockenden[68] in 1968,
where the 'villas' were all named after trees.
There we were taught the medical definitions
of 'idiot', of 'imbecile',
and of 'moral imbecile'.
And we were shown examples of each type.
My four weeks of psychiatry undergraduate training
was full of fascinating strangeness.

---

[67] The Aymara are an indigenous group with a rich heritage living in the Andes and Altiplano of Bolivia and Peru.
[68] South Ockenden Hospital in Essex, known locally as 'The Colony', was a long-stay institution for patients with severe learning disabilities which closed in 1994.

198.

Among 'the undesirables' at South Ockendon,
there were some working inmates
who seemed unimpaired.
There were also murderers,
like John Straffen[69],
who was contained
in the guarded Cypress facility.
What I saw that day
had a far greater impact on my training
than any lecture.

---

[69] John Straffen (1930-2007) was a notorious brain-damaged child murderer who at the time of his death was Britain's longest serving prisoner, incarcerated for 55 years.

R. THE OLD MASTERS

199.
Anyone interested
in functional neurological disorder
needs to read all Charcot's[70] later writings
on hysteria.
And the ideas of his late collaborator,
Pierre Janet[71].

200.
Charcot outlined the territory
for the future speciality of neurology,
then got the opportunity
to capture hysteria from the alienists,
who were then left to care for the insane,
the demented,
and the mentally impaired.
As far as the lucrative neuroses were concerned,
it remained a free-for-all.

---

[70] Jean-Martin Charcot (1825-1893) was a Parisian physician who is now regarded as the founding father of neurology.
[71] Pierre Janet (1859-1947) was a French medical psychologist who contributed greatly to the understanding of hysteria, dissociated states and traumatic childhood memory.

201.

Christopher Earl[72],

one of my teachers at Queen Square,

told me that

it was better I try to find things out myself

than take someone else's word for it.

Like many of my teachers,

he encouraged me

to question things.

202.

Dr Gooddy[73] told me

that his boss Frances Walshe

once told him,

'Neuroscience was the triumph

of technique over reason'.

Now you understand how I ended up

a sceptic and a flaneur.

---

[72] Christopher Earl (1925-2012) was a British neurologist on the staff at the National Hospital and the Middlesex Hospital and one of my favourite teachers.
[73] William Gooddy (1916-2004) was British neurologist on the staff of the National Hospital, Queen Square and University College Hospital, London who encouraged me to read Proust and take an interest in Time and the nervous system.

203.

I encountered monstrous diva doctors
who inspired loyalty and devotion
and even heartfelt love.
They had cast iron probity
and a certain greatness.
They were arrogant,
but they were far better
than the insipid 'Suits you sir,
Anything for a quiet life' type
that has replaced them.

204.

Of the greats at Queen Square,
David Ferrier[74] was the least spoken about.
Perhaps because his main contributions
related to animal research.
I was always intrigued
by his joint appointment at King's,
in what is now called forensic pathology.

---

[74] David Ferrier (1843-1928) was a Scottish neurologist who
worked at the National Hospital, Queen Square in London and
carried out pioneering preclinical work on localisation in the
cerebral cortex.

205.

I am a 'back of an envelope'
or 'front of a beer mat' clinical neuroscientist,
like my former colleague David Marsden[75].

206.

Gheorghe Marinescu[76],
Romanian neurologist and pathologist,
played a key role
behind the scenes
through collaborations with Blocq and Brissaud,
And with his Russian student Tretiakoff,
in identifying loss of pars compacta nigral neurones
as the pathological substrate
for Parkinson's disease.

---

[75] C. David Marsden (1938-1998) was the leading clinical neuroscientist of his generation who worked first at Kings College Hospital and the Institute of Psychiatry before taking the Chair of Neurology at the Institute of Neurology, Queen Square in 1987.
[76] Gheorghe Marinescu (1863-1938) was the Founder of Romanian neurology after postgraduate studies in Paris with Charcot and Marie, and Weigert in Frankfurt.

207.
Gowers Manual[77] and Charcot's *Oeuvres Complètes*[78]
are the best treatises on neurology.
While both men knew the medical literature,
their written accounts come primarily
from their own observations and experience.

208.
I find it disappointing
that the role of my mentor Gerald Stern[79]
in founding Parkinsons UK in 1970,
together with Mali Jenkins,
the sister of one of his patients,
has been rubbed out
from the charity's annals.

---

[77] *A Manual of Diseases of the Nervous System* by William Gowers, a
two-volume work published in 1886 and 1888.
[78] *Oeuvres Complètes de J-M Charcot*, published 1887.
[79] Gerald Stern (1930-2018) was a British neurologist on the staff of
University College Hospital, London and my most important
mentor.

209.

Macdonald Critchley[80] was fascinated
by silent language.
He learned the bookmakers' language of tick-tack
and taught me a few of the signs
in his home at Queen's Court.

210.

Listening to my teachers Gerald Stern
and Christopher Earl
teach me neurology
often felt like walking through surf
and letting the sea bathe my bare feet.
Then if they showed me how to elicit a sign,
I was riding the waves.

---

[80] Macdonald Critchley (1900-1997) was a British neurologist on
the staff of the National Hospital, Queen Square.

211.
Madman[81] is about clinical research,
Brainspotting[82] about practice.
Gowers, Charcot, Wilson, Critchley,
Adams[83], Miller Fisher[84] and many more
managed to excel in both.
There is still a place in medicine
for the curious practitioner.

212.
Robert Schwab,
who gave evidence in the Jack Ruby case,
could reasonably be considered,
along with Kinnier Wilson and Rolf Hassler,
as one of the most important
Parkinson's clinical researchers.
He has always been one of my remote influences.

---

[81] *Mentored by a Madman: The William Burroughs Experiment* (Notting Hill Editions), published in 2017.
[82] *Brainspotting: Adventures in Neurology* (Notting Hill Editions) published in 2022.
[83] Raymond Adams (1911-2008) was an American neurologist and neuropathologist and head of Massachusetts General Hospital in Boston.
[84] C Miller Fisher (1913-2012) was a Canadian neurologist who made a huge contribution to the clinical pathological understanding of stroke.

213.

Neurology textbooks are worth reading,
but only the old ones —
Gowers manual.
Charcot-Lecons du Mardi.
Matthews'[85] Practical Neurology.
Patten[86].
And Harry Lee Parker[87].

214.

The anatomo-clinical method,
physiological advances,
and David Ferrier's animal studies
underpinned the emergence of neurology in Britain.

215.

Laycock's students in York and Edinburgh,
the West Riding Lunatic asylum,
Brown-Sequard, Jackson,
Bastian and Gowers,
all working at Queen Square,
set the stage
for the speciality of neurology in Great Britain.

---

[85] Bryan Matthews (1906-1986) was a Professor of Neurology at Oxford University.
[86] John Patten was a British neurologist and author of *Neurological Differential Diagnosis*.
[87] Harry Lee Parker (1894-1959) was an Irish American neurologist and author of *Clinical Studies in Neurology*.

216.
Why did William Gowers
emphasise the value
of shorthand (phonography)
in clinical practice?
Because he knew
that the words his patients used
were diagnostic distress calls.
His descriptions of disease
come directly from his detailed case histories.
Always keep your own case notes,
even if it takes extra time.

217.
I agree with Pascal
that it is not possible
to have a reasonable belief
against miracles or catastrophes.

218.
One can discern Pascal's two threads of thought
within the history of neurology.
The analytical always holding sway,
but the intuitive never quite going away.
Some of my teachers
could smell mischief.

219.

When I did laboratory work
in the Curzon[88] lab in '79,
I realised that scientific research
was arduous and painstaking.
I learned to acknowledge my ignorance
and be sceptical.
It was completely different
than training to be a physician.

220.

My advice to young neurologists:
Neither a leader nor a follower be.
Be a light unto yourself.
Always check your sources.
Question everything.
Always remember the neurological literature
began with Thomas Willis[89],
and not in 2000
with Aaron Aaronson[90].

---

[88] Gerald Curzon (1928-2019) was Professor of Neurochemistry at the Institute of Neurology, Queen Square, London who had a particular interest in brain serotonin.

[89] Thomas Willis (1621-1675) was an English physician who coined the term 'neurology' and did some pioneering research on the anatomy of the human brain.

[90] A joke which relates back to the time when some science journals listed the small list of authors in alphabetical order leading to some

221.
The notion of 'other ways, other times'
is foreign to modern multiculturalists,
who are certain
that 'they know best'.
All that came before
was atavistic and inconsequential.

222.
The doctor-patient interaction
is pure drama.
And the best neurological teachers like Charcot
have a natural theatricality
and way with words,
which is very different
from the self-congratulatory showmanship
of mediocre diva doctors.
Critchley[91] always wanted to go on stage,
and Jonathan Miller[92] did.

---

heads of department allegedly using pseudonyms beginning with two letter a's.
[91] MacDonald Critchley (1900-1997) was an English Neurologist who worked at the National Hospital, Queen Square, London.
[92] Jonathan Miller (1934-2019) was an English theatre and opera director, actor and comedian who qualified as a doctor and had some regrets he had not pursued a career in neurology.

S. Parkinson's Disease

223.
One of my patient's told me
that she had discovered a new visual cue
to overcome blocking of gait.
This involved closing her eyes
and visualising an empty beach.

224.
The study of Parkinson's disease dream content
has always been of great interest to me.
We need more personal accounts,
and not just the auguries
or those reporting restored movement in dreams.

225.

To discontinue L-DOPA and oral dopamine agonists
perioperatively
and replace them with a rotigotine[93] skin patch
is dangerous for people with Parkinsons disease
who have had major bowel surgery
and are nil by mouth.
By far the safest approach
is the use of a subcutaneous apomorphine[94] pump.

226.

'Soft Parkinsonian signs' in the elderly
are much more likely due to tau[95] accumulation
in the brain
or to cerebrovascular pathology
than to nigral[96] cell loss and Lewy pathology.

---

[93] A medication used to treat Parkinson's disease which binds to
dopamine receptors in the brain.
[94] A dopamine analogue used to treat Parkinson's disease.
[95] Tau proteins are abundant in the human brain and are
important in maintaining the transport system along axons.
[96] Relating to the substantia nigra in the midbrain, a group of
pigmented nerve cells that are damaged in Parkinson's disease.

227.

The hypotensive 'twilight zone'
is important and common in Parkinson's disease
and under-recognised by neurologists.
It can take different forms,
including feeling unwell, fuzzy headedness,
and even momentary unrousability when sitting.

228.

Why is reduced alpha synuclein[97]
not pathogenic to the brain?
Why has synuclein replacement been dismissed
without being tested?
Answer: it does not suit the scientific zeitgeist.

229.

The 1960s and 70s
were a golden therapeutic age.
All the most efficacious types
of Parkinsons disease medications
are at least 50 years old.
These treatments are vastly superior
to anything molecular biology has come up with
for any of the common neurodegenerations.

---

[97] Alpha synuclein is a protein involved in the regulation and release of brain neurotransmitters. Pathological aggregation of synuclein due to misfolding of the protein is widely believed to be the cause of Parkinson's disease.

230.

Apomorphine is a dopamine analogue
with similar pharmacological properties to L-DOPA.
When administered under the skin using a pump,
there is no evidence
that it is more likely to produce impulse control behaviour
or hallucinations,
than L-DOPA[98] formulations.

231.

Parkinson's disease can begin suddenly
after a severe emotional shock,
usually with tremor.
This can lead to misdiagnosis
as a psychogenic movement disorder
and may be accompanied by unjustified guilt
in family members if they believe they were responsible.

232.

Clues to emerging cognitive impairment
in Parkinson's disease:
reversible post-operative delirium.
Vagueness.
Abulia[99].
Frightening visual hallucinations.
Daytime somnolence.
Fuzzy vision.

---

[98] A naturally occurring amino acid and pro-drug which is
converted in the brain to the chemical messenger dopamine.
[99] Abulia is loss of willpower and capacity to act decisively.

233.
It's good news week.
Selegiline[100] is back.
But now rasagiline has disappeared.
Of the two,
I have always found selegiline more efficacious,
but both are superior
to the more expensive safinamide.

234.
Massive publicity this week in the UK
for fos-levodopa,
a treatment with very limited data.
Not one mention of the fact
that subcutaneous pump therapy
has been available for Parkinsons disease
for 35 years.
The long arm of Pharma at work.

235.
If one had to choose
between only using the anti-Parkinsonian medications
developed before 1990
and those developed in the last 30 years,
it would be judged a no-contest.
And yet the old ones keep going missing.

---

[100] Selegiline was the first marketed monoamine oxidase B
inhibitor for the treatment of Parkinson's disease, and rasagiline
and safinamide are more recent ones. In the UK it has disappeared
periodically to the detriment of patients' care.

T. Research

236.

Other New England Journal[101] gaffes
in Parkinson's disease
were the 2001 DBS STN[102] trial,
which nefariously underreported dysarthria
and the 2023 FUS[103] pallidotomy trial,
whose results were historically inferior
to radiofrequency pallidal lesions
but hyped in the discussion.

237.

Statistics, damned statistics!
Remember the importance of the Reverend Bayes
in determining medical probability and meaningfulness.
Too many lacunes in our knowledge
of the course of Alzheimer's and Parkinson's disease
to be excited about small statistical differences.

---

[101] The prestigious *New England Journal of Medicine* has made a series
of poor judgements in relation to acceptance of research with
accompanying effusive editorials on Parkinson's disease that have
been proved subsequently to be misjudgements.
[102] Abbreviations for Deep Brain Stimulation of the Subthalamic
Nuclei, a widely used surgical procedure.
[103] Functional ultrasound therapy is a new approach to surgical
treatment for tremor and Parkinson's disease.

238.

The study of a person and their diseases
can be looked upon as an unrepeatable n=1 experiment.
But what is discovered
can become a medical metaphor.
It is not science.

239.

The Heisenberg Uncertainty Principle[104]
could be used to hypothesise
that the more precisely
the pathology of a disease is determined,
the less exactly the clinical implications are known.

240.

Much of science is occult.
It grew out of magic,
not Greek philosophy.
Which is why I believe
everything happens for a reason,
and why the word 'stochastic'
seems inappropriate and opaque.

---

[104] Heisenberg Uncertainty Principle is a concept in quantum
mechanics which states that there is a limit to the precision with
which certain pairs of physical properties can be simultaneously
known: the more one is measured, the less accurately the other can
be understood.

241.

Are there any practitioners
who believe that medicine
is a life science?
Medicine is, and always has been,
an art underpinned by scientific facts
and by clinical experience.
I see this basic misconception as contributing
to the angst clinical neuroscience
has got itself into.

242.

Are there any organs in the human body
where abnormal aggregation of alpha synuclein
has been looked for in late-stage Parkinson's disease
and not been found?

243.

I've just been reviewing the latest papers on Bell's palsy[105].
It is remarkable how little we still know
about its causation and course.
And how devoid the medical literature is
of descriptions of the challenges of living
with residual facial weakness
and a crooked smile.

---

[105] Sudden onset of weakness of the whole of one side of the face
due to facial nerve paralysis. It is of uncertain cause but usually
recovers over weeks to months.

244.

Perhaps we should not blame Braak or Frau Braak
or Kelly Tredici or Chris Hawkes
but instead the neurologists, pathologists and scientists
who accepted the Braak hypothesis[106] uncritically.
It filled a gap
and generated synuclein grants,
but none designed to prove or refute it.

245.

In the 1970's,
it was estimated
that there were 50,000 people
with Parkinsons disease in UK.
The figure quoted is now 153,000.
Life expectancy has improved,
and the population has grown,
but I am sceptical
that underdiagnosis
or misdiagnosis
are important additional explanations.

---

[106] The Braak hypothesis proposes that the pathological process of
Parkinson's disease begins in the gut and olfactory bulb and then
progresses to the medulla oblongata in the central nervous system
and ascends through the brain stem to the cerebral cortex.

U. Shifting Paradigms

246.

How much easier it was
as a medical student
to shut oneself in the library
than to visit the wards,
but as time went on,
I realised I was gleaning far more by the 'doing'
than the passive absorption of facts.
My textbooks are passé,
but I can picture those first patients clearly.

247.

I have come to find borderland specialities
both essential and fascinating.
Neuro-gastroenterology
is the latest to establish itself.
Neuro-orthopaedics needs nurturing.

248.

It was Charcot who proposed the name
'Maladie de Parkinson'
as preferable to paralysis agitans.
One hundred and fifty years on,
there are peacockian colleagues
who want to rub out the disease Parkinson described
and replace it
with the name of a protein.

249.

The blinkered acceptance of Braak's hypothesis
has set back creative thinking on Parkinson's disease.
The gut first/ brain first dichotomy[107],
based on imaging studies,
is of the same ilk
and even more fanciful.
Both ignore nerve cell loss
in the brain and periphery.

---

[107] The gut first, brain first hypothesis proposes that the
pathological process responsible for Parkinson's disease can start
either in the enteric nervous system of the gut or in the brain with
each having a distinct pathway of progression.

250.

The severest and commonest sign of Parkinson's disease
is due to nerve cell loss
in the ventrolateral tier of the pars compacta
of the substantia nigra.
It has nothing to do with alpha synuclein aggregation.
That recurrent ugly little fact
that keeps getting in the way.

251.

We need to nurture physicians
who can deal with any neurological symptom.
And we need more clinics
where specialists from different medical disciplines
work together.
An overabundance of sub-specialists
at the expense of generalists
is not healthy.

252.

In relation to treatments for Parkinsons disease,
I remain enthusiastic
about the physiological restoration
of striatal[108] dopamine.
About ethnobotanical exploration.
And about holistic autotherapy.
We have also barely scratched the surface
in our understanding
of the role of nicotine and stress.

253.

'Fission fusion' medical societies
never provide the cohesion,
the sustained mentorship,
or the safe anchoring
that came with medical apprenticeship
and attachment to a medical or surgical firm,
even when there was no long-term security.

---

[108] Striatal refers to the corpus striatum, a region of the basal
ganglia rich in dopamine that plays a role in movement, decision
making and pleasure and reward.

254.

Abolition of the medical firm system[109].
No place for papyrus,
no location to talk to relatives,
or to confer with colleagues.
More meaningless metrics
pointless scales,
disease mongering,
and overdiagnosis.

255.

Tell me,
where are those doctors
who you knew so well in their lifetime,
in the full flowering of their learning?
Other men now sit in their seats.
The old masters are hardly ever called to mind.
In their lifetime they seemed of great account.
Now, no one speaks of them.

---

[109] A model of medical training and patient care where groups of
doctors under the guidance of a senior doctor provide care and
learn from each other.

256.

I can't work out
whether more juniors are mumbling
in grand round presentations due to shyness
or even a desire to be misunderstood.
Or whether I am increasingly hard of hearing.
But microphones seem to be being used more,
even in small lecture theatres.

257.

Perhaps like many other physicians in England
I now feel more venerable
when I am called doc. rather than prof.
Professors were once distinguished by scholarship,
but now the term does not distinguish
between careerist and bureaucrat,
nor between academic entrepreneur and intellectual.

V. SOULFUL NEUROLOGY

258.
What's wrong with melodrama?
What's wrong with saudade[110]?
What's wrong with sobbing?
What's wrong with 'all for one and one for all'?

259.
Imagine there's a ward round.
It's easy if you try.
Imagine there's a story
far more diagnostic than a test.
Hold this book in your hands,
read the words out loud,
pop it in the pocket
of a white coat.
Birdsong for the attuned.

---

[110] A recurrent feeling of longing, yearning and melancholy that is integral to Lusitanians.

260.

Every time you go out
and sit with a book in a café,
listen to what is being said around you.
And look what is going on,
all your senses on full alert.
Look for intersections with your patients.
This is a neglected facet
of the clinical method.

261.

When I open the doors to my heart,
I become a soulful neurologist.
When the cardiac chambers slam shut,
I am A.J. Lees,
and no use to anyone.

262.

In this Nietzschean[111] age,
I find I am drawn more
to the powerless and insubordinate person
on the street.
I am attracted to Soho cafes,
where one can strike up a conversation
about an inconsequential topic
with a total stranger.

---

[111] Friedrich Nietzsche (1844-1900) was a German philosopher.

263.
Barely a day goes by
without me seeing someone
with an abnormal movement disorder
in the street
or on the Tube.
Only a minority will ever be seen
in a neurology clinic.
More will be seen by mental health services,
drug rehabilitation clinics,
and day centres for the elderly.

264.
Sometimes coming home on the Tube,
a diagnosis, which had eluded me in clinic,
beams in.

265.
I used to dislike
Tottenham Court Road station.
But it is one of my favourites now.
I link it with akathisia[112],
with carrier bags full of old books
and with Essex.

---

[112] Akathisia is a neuropsychiatric disorder seen mostly in people receiving antipsychotic medication and characterised by an inability to sit still with continuous movements like marching on the spot or aimless walking.

266.

Northern line,
linked with seizures and the suburbs.
People look resigned
and devoid of hope.
A disturbed impulsive hyperactive child
leading his mother on a dance.

267.

Has anybody seen a proper tramp recently?
I am referring to a professional vagabond
who loves the open road,
the scent of nature,
and the freedom of penury.
CCTV has driven them from the cities,
but I am hoping a few survive,
walking the country lanes.

268.

Sometimes during my flânerie,
I decide to take the first right,
then the first left,
then the first right,
and so on.
It is a fascinating way
of observing the human zoo.

W. Synuclein Testing

269.
The severity of bradykinesia correlates
with the degree of ventral nigral cell loss
and not with Lewy pathology.
So how can synuclein measurement
be considered the lynchpin
for a biological definition
of maladie de Parkinson?
In isolation it is not even enough
to fulfil the pathological definition.

270.
I see the alpha synuclein seed amplification assay
as a test of comparable usefulness
to the dopamine transporter SPECT scan
in the diagnosis of Parkinson's disease.
It will be attractive to insecure clinicians
and to private practitioners.

271.

I can imagine
that the diagnosis will be explained
by the craftless hyposkilliacs[113],
without discussion of the symptoms
or mention of the pathognomonic signs,
as if the redundant dopamine transporter scan
or the synuclein blood test
was the final arbiter.

272.

Many of those promoting the widespread use
of amyloid, tau and synuclein seed assays
behave like salespeople
talking to consumers.
They do not provide cogent arguments.
Reminds me of the war on Iraq.

273.

The alpha synuclein and tau seed amplification assays
do not replace the clinical diagnosis of Parkinson's disease.
But they may be of some use
in aiding the early differentiation of PSP-P
from Parkinson's disease
and some other rare non-Lewy body disorders.

---

[113] A term coined by the cardiologist Dr H.L Fred to describe a
deficiency of clinical skills in a physician.

274.
What I see coming,
based on what has happened in Alzheimer's disease,
is a lot of older folk with pseudo-Parkinsonism
and a positive synuclein test
being put on L-DOPA,
to which they will have no response
and some adverse reactions.
Let us stop this
before it happens.

275.
I refuse to be forced to use synuclein seed assays
in clinical trials in Parkinson's disease
without more debate.
Neuronal synuclein disease[114]
is a clinically irrelevant term
that needs swatting.

---

[114] A pathological term used to describe a group of disorders which have an abnormal accumulation of alpha synuclein protein in the brain.

276.

The proponents of the seed assay[115]
and of neuronal synucleinopathy,
will dismiss the Masliah scandal
as just the exposure of an outlying rogue scientist
instead of considering what it means
to the credibility of their proposals.

277.

Based on the data in 2024,
the only rational conclusion
is that the synuclein test
is of extremely limited value
in clinical practice.
Even less than a DAT scan.
As a research test,
combined with other biomarkers,
it is of great interest.

---

[115] The alpha synuclein seed amplification assay is a laboratory test used to identify misfolded protein aggregates. Its clinical usefulness remains to be determined.

278.

Early distinction between Parkinson's disease
and atypical Parkinsonism
is the greatest challenge in diagnosis.
Synuclein pathology is found
in 20% of PSP[116] and CBD[117] cases.
And the alpha synuclein assay's inability also
to accurately distinguish MSA[118] from PD
makes the test of negligible clinical value for now.
It is a research test.

279.

Asymptomatic elderly people
should not be screened with biomarkers
for Alzheimer's or Parkinson's disease.
The harm far outweighs any possible early pick up.
In recent years I have seen dementia overdiagnosis.
It is a serious iatrogenic disorder
which needs stamping on.

---

[116] Progressive supranuclear palsy is a neurodegenerative disorder characterised by an inability to look down, poor balance leading to falls backwards, signs of Parkinsonism, frontal lobe and pseudobulbar signs.
[117] Corticobasal degeneration is a rare neurodegenerative disorder characterised by a jerky dystonic 'useless' alien limb, slurred speech, focal cognitive decline and muscular stiffness.
[118] Multiple system atrophy is a neurodegenerative disorder characterised by early severe failure of the autonomic nervous system, unsteadiness, slurred speech, bradykinesia and rigidity. It is often difficult to distinguish in the early stages from Parkinsons disease.

X. Wanderlust

280.

During my stage in Paris,
I read the *Leçons du Mardi*[119]
in the Charcot library.
It was like first reading a detective novel
and then being able to see
In the *Nouvelle Iconographie de la Salpêtrière*[120],
daguerreotypes of the victims.

281.

When I go to Paris,
I want a grand crème,
not a Latte
or a Cappuccino.
When I want a light lunch,
I want *une omelette aux fines herbes*,
not a cheeseburger.
I also prefer the customary surly service.

---

[119] A series of clinical lectures delivered by Jean Martin Charcot at
the Salpêtrière Hospital in Paris.
[120] French medical journal published from 1888-1918 featuring
many photographs and drawings of nervous disease.

282.
Sometimes over the years on day trips to Paris,
I have spent more than half the time
travelling the Metropolitan
exploring new stations and vistas.

283.
Since I started to visit Brazil in 1984,
the country has teetered
between light and dark.

284.
I feel closer to Cuba than I have in years.
PayPal blocks me buying its coffee,
and the world's bullies are waiting
to turn the world's largest sofa
into Sunset Strip.
The Cubans I know are musical people.

Y. Wearable Technology

285.
Attempts to develop
simple wearable gadgets
to aid walking and speaking,
balance and dyskinesias,
continue apace.
Short observational studies
by impartial and skilled investigators
in randomly selected volunteers
are feasible and essential.

286.
Can anyone give me an example
where a wearable, a gadget, or a scale,
has provided data in Parkinson's disease
that could not be obtained
by history taking
and by a focused neurological examination?
Or which changed treatment?

287.

I'm trying to imagine a scenario
of a neurologist explaining
to a patient complaining of increased slowness
around 4 in the afternoon
that they are imagining it,
because the wearable shows
that they have improved.

288.

The kindling of health anxiety
is highly profitable.
For a healthy person,
monitoring 24-hour glucose
is a ridiculous waste of money
that should never be funded.
Next will be a MoCa[121] or MMSE[122] administered daily,
with the amyloid blood test[123] once a year.
Call it out.

---

[121] The Montreal Cognitive Assessment is a brief test of cognition used to screen for dementia.
[122] The Mini Mental State Examination is a brief, eleven-question measure to test five areas of cognitive function.
[123] Lumipulse G. pTau217/ß-Amyloid 1-42 plasma ratio blood test for the early detection of amyloid plaques associated with Alzheimer's disease.

289.

What you can measure
in Parkinsons disease
with costly gadgets
and cluttering wearables
is of negligible value.
A history and examination
with a competent neurologist
lasting 45 minutes
twice a year
is what is needed.

Z. Writing

290.
A situation has arrived.
The Royal Mail,
with a history going back
to the seventeenth century
and a loved institution by my generation,
is now dependent on rescue
by a Tech billionaire.
Write letters and post cards using a pen
to friends who can cherish them forever.

291.
Authors should 'caress' the figures included in their papers
with a few words of explanation
embedded in the body of the text,
and not rely only on a legend.
In that way,
the reader understands the rationale
for the legend's inclusion
and the points it is trying to emphasise.

292.

Many scientists deliberately write
in a way that the less their readership understand,
the cleverer it will think them to be —
rather like a Latin Mass.

293.

Much of the psychological literature
is riddled with jargon,
cleverly designed
to create an illusion
that something profound has been written.
The canon casts a long shadow
over the English language.

294.

My father taught me
that literary style
was simply having something of interest to say
and expressing it clearly.
That's where medicine's recent love
for municipal decorated gothic
comes a cropper.

295.

Sloppy hyperbolic cliché-ridden language
combined with jargon, acronyms and abbreviation
devoid of basic rules of grammar
makes for tepid reading.
Plain Words by Ernest Gowers —
a good place for everyone to start.

296.

I would much rather my books were not translated
than accept second-rate machine translation.
I need to be sure too
that my translator knows the subject
and understands the necessity for nuance.
'Avaricious' is not the same as 'bloody greedy'.

297.

In my heart,
I only remember my childhood.
Nothing else truly belongs to me.
To understand my writing,
you need to understand what the world
and my life
were like
when I was 18.

298.
Much of my writing
consists of adverse criticism of this life.
Some may consider it self-indulgent
and a misuse of literary privilege.
But I hope that,
through grousing,
I can speak for those
who cannot speak for themselves.
And evoke magic moments
from the verbiage.

299.
Migraine and *Awakenings*
are Oliver Sacks' greatest books,
because they are authentic —
like the Beatles' first two albums.
The Man who Mistook his Wife for a Hat
is his worst.
Yet it is the one that brought so many bright minds
into neurology.

300.
There is a need for a new book on neurology
written by a master clinician
who has spent most of her life taking medical histories.
It needs to be rich in anecdotes
and to focus on symptoms.
It should detail the tried and tested clinical pearls
and the diagnostic tips
that have been passed down by oral tradition.
And then list the likely causes
on the basis of their probability.

www.ingramcontent.com/pod-product-compliance
Lightning Source LLC
Chambersburg PA
CBHW032112280326
41933CB00009B/807